Mediterr- DIE Cookbook 2021

Easy, Flavorful Mediterranean Diet Recipes for Lifelong Health!.

Angela D. Lovato

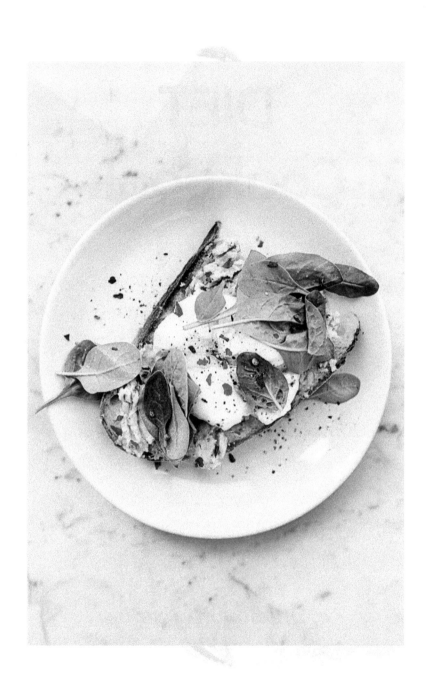

Table of content

MEDITERRANEAN BREAKFAST RECIPE

PAXIMADIA

Makes 36

- 3 large eggs, beaten
- 1 1⁄2 cups vegetable oil
- 1 1⁄2 cups sugar
- 2 teaspoons vanilla extract
- 1 teaspoon almond extract
- 4 cups all-purpose flour
- 1 teaspoon baking powder
- 1 cup chopped almonds
- 1 cup sesame seeds

Directions

- Preheat the oven to 350°F. In a large bowl, whisk together eggs, oil, sugar, and extracts. Combine the flour, baking powder, and almonds and then stir the mixture into the wet ingredients until it forms a soft dough.
- Divide the dough and form three equal loaves (9" × 3"). Place equal amounts of the sesame seeds on three pieces of wax paper. Wrap the paper around each loaf so the sesame seeds coat the entire loaf. Repeat with the remaining loaves.
- Place the loaves on a parchment paper–lined baking sheet. Bake on the middle rack for 20 minutes. Take the baking sheet out of the oven and reduce the temperature to 300°F.

- Cool the loaves for 2 minutes. Slice each loaf along its width into 3⁄4-inch slices with a serrated knife. Lay the slices flat on the baking sheet and
- bake them for another 10 minutes. Turn off the oven, but leave the paximadia in the oven for another 30 minutes.
- Store in a sealed container for up to 6 months.

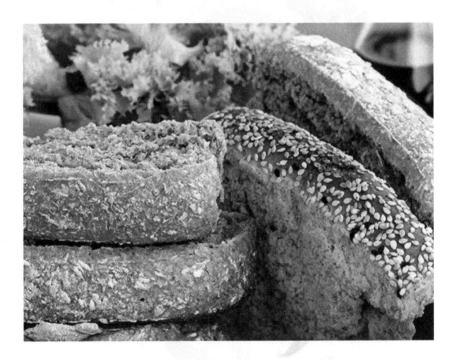

LENTEN PAXIMADIA

These paximadia are perfect for fasting during Lent because there are no eggs in this recipe.

Makes 36

- 1⁄2 cup fresh orange juice
- 1 tablespoon grated orange zest
- 3⁄4 cup vegetable oil
- 1⁄2 cup dry white wine
- 11⁄2 teaspoons ground cinnamon
- 1⁄4 teaspoon ground cloves
- 3⁄4 cup sugar
- 1⁄4 teaspoon baking soda
- 11⁄2 tablespoons baking powder 1 cup chopped almonds
- 3 cups all-purpose flour
- 1 cup sesame seeds

Directions

- Preheat the oven to 350°F. Add the orange juice, zest, oil, wine, cinnamon, cloves, sugar, baking soda, and baking powder to a food processor and process until the ingredients are well incorporated. In a large bowl, stir together the almonds and flour. Pour the orange juice mixture into the flour mixture and, using a wooden spoon, combine until it forms a soft dough.
- Divide the dough and form three equal loaves (9" × 3"). Place equal amounts of sesame seeds on three pieces of wax paper. Wrap the paper around each loaf so the

sesame seeds coat the entire loaf. Repeat with the remaining loaves.

- Place the loaves on a parchment paper–lined baking sheet. Bake on the middle rack for 20 minutes. Take the baking sheet out of the oven and reduce the oven to 300°F.

- Cool the loaves for 2 minutes. Slice each loaf along its width into 3⁄4-inch slices with a serrated knife. Lay the slices flat on the baking sheet, and bake them for another 10 minutes. Turn off the oven, but leave the paximadia in the oven for another 30 minutes.

- Store them in a sealed container for up to 6 months.

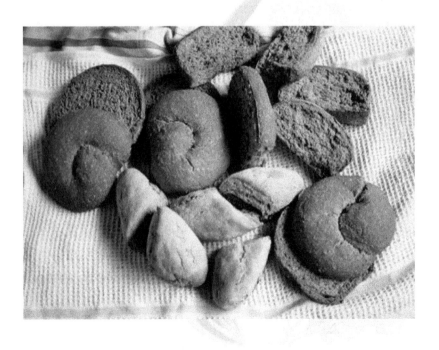

PAXIMADIA WITH FIGS, STAR ANISE, AND WALNUTS

Star anise is a spice that is similar to anise, but it has a more floral scent and taste.

Serves 36

- 1 cup extra-virgin olive oil
- 2 teaspoons vanilla extract
- 4 tablespoons ground star anise
- 1 ounce ouzo
- 1 cup sugar
- 3 large eggs
- 4 cups all-purpose flour
- 1 tablespoon baking powder
- 1 cup chopped dry figs
- 1 cup chopped walnuts
- 2 tablespoons petimezi (grape molasses) diluted in 2 tablespoons warm water 1 cup sesame seeds

Directions

- In a large bowl, whisk together oil, vanilla, star anise, ouzo, sugar, and eggs. In another bowl, combine the flour, baking powder, figs, and walnuts. Add the dry ingredients to the wet ingredients. Use a wooden spoon to combine the mixture until you form a soft dough.
- Divide the dough and form three equal loaves (9" × 3"). Brush the tops of the loaves with the petimezi mixture. Place equal amounts of sesame seeds on three pieces of

wax paper. Wrap a sheet of paper around each loaf so the sesame seeds coat the entire loaf. Repeat with the remaining loaves.

- Place the loaves on a parchment paper–lined baking sheet. Bake them on the middle rack for 20 minutes. Take the baking sheet out of the oven and reduce the oven to 300°F.

- Cool the loaves for 2 minutes. Slice each loaf along its width into 3⁄4-inch slices with a serrated knife. Lay the slices flat on the baking sheet and bake for another 10 minutes. Turn off the oven, but leave the paximadia in the oven for another 30 minutes.

- Store in a sealed container for up to 6 months.

BOUGATSA WITH CUSTARD FILLING

Serves 12

- 2 cups melted unsalted butter, divided
- 3⁄4 cup fine semolina flour
- 1⁄2 cup granulated sugar
- 1 teaspoon vanilla extract
- 23⁄4 cups whole milk
- 24 sheets phyllo (1 package)
- 1⁄2 cup confectioners' sugar
- 2 teaspoons ground cinnamon

Directions

- In a deep, medium pot over medium heat, add 1⁄4 cup butter, semolina, sugar, and vanilla. Stir and cook for 2 minutes or until the butter is absorbed and the semolina is golden but not browned.
- Whisk in milk in a slow, steady stream until all the liquid is absorbed. Stir and cook for 3–4 minutes or until the custard has the texture of loose cream. Transfer the custard to a bowl and allow it to cool completely.
- Preheat oven to 350°F. Take phyllo sheets out of the box and lay them flat. Cover with a lightly damp kitchen towel to keep them from drying out. You will work with one sheet at a time. Keep the remaining sheets covered. Take one phyllo sheet and lay it on a clean work surface; brush the phyllo with melted butter and cover it with another phyllo sheet.

14

- Brush the top of the second phyllo sheet with butter as well.
- Place 3 tablespoons of custard in the center bottom third of the buttered phyllo sheets (about 2 inches from the edge). Fold the bottom 2 inches over the custard, and then fold the sides in toward the custard. Fold the phyllo up to form a package. Repeat with the remaining phyllo and custard.
- Bake the phyllo packages on a baking sheet for 15–20 minutes or until golden. Allow them to cool. Dust them with confectioners' sugar and cinnamon before serving.

FIG, APRICOT, AND ALMOND GRANOLA

Serves 16

- Nonstick vegetable oil spray
- 1/3 cup vegetable oil
- 1/3 cup honey
- 2 tablespoons white sugar
- 1 teaspoon vanilla extract
- 4 cups old-fashioned oats
- 1 1/4 cups sliced almonds
- 1/2 cup chopped dried apricots
- 1/2 cup chopped dried figs
- 1/2 cup (packed) brown sugar
- 1/2 teaspoon salt
- 1/2 teaspoon ground cardamom

Directions

- Preheat the oven to 300°F. Lightly spray two large baking sheets with nonstick spray.
- In a small pot over medium heat, add oil, honey, sugar, and vanilla. Cook for 5 minutes or until the sugar is dissolved. Remove the pot from the heat and let it cool for 2 minutes.
- In a large bowl, combine oats, almonds, apricots, figs, brown sugar, salt, and cardamom. Mix with your hands to combine.
- Pour the hot liquid over the dry ingredients. Using your hands (if it is too hot, use a wooden spoon), toss the

ingredients together to make sure everything is well coated. Spread the granola evenly over two baking sheets. Bake for 30 minutes (stirring every 10 minutes).

- Let the granola cool completely on the baking sheets. This will allow the granola to harden before breaking it up into pieces. Store in an airtight container for up to 3 weeks.

MEDITERRANEAN
LUNCH RECIPE

Mediterranean Edamame Toss

Ingredients

- ½ cup uncooked quinoa, rinsed and drained
- 1 cup water
- 1 cup ready-to-eat fresh or frozen, thawed shelled sweet soybeans (edamame)
- 2 medium tomatoes, seeded and chopped
- 1 cup fresh arugula or spinach leaves
- ½ cup chopped red onion
- 2 tablespoons olive oil
- 1 teaspoon finely shredded lemon peel
- 2 tablespoons lemon juice
- ¼ cup crumbled reduced-fat feta cheese
- 2 tablespoons snipped fresh basil
- ¼ teaspoon salt
- ¼ teaspoon freshly ground black pepper

Directions

- In a medium saucepan, combine quinoa and water. Bring to boiling; reduce heat. Cover and simmer about 15 minutes or until quinoa is tender and liquid is absorbed, adding edamame the last 4 minutes of cooking.
- In a large bowl, combine quinoa mixture, tomato, arugula, and onion.
- In a small bowl, whisk together olive oil, lemon peel, and lemon juice. Stir in half of the cheese, the basil, salt, and pepper. Add mixture to quinoa mixture, tossing to coat.

Sprinkle with remaining half of the cheese. Serve at room temperature.

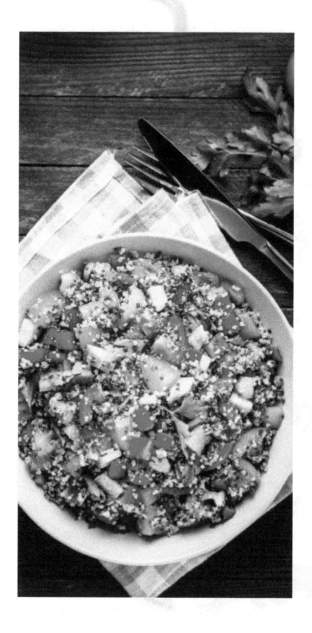

Fig & Goat Cheese Salad

Ingredients

- 2 cups mixed salad greens
- 4 dried figs, stemmed and sliced
- 1 ounce fresh goat cheese, crumbled
- 1 ½ tablespoons slivered almonds, preferably toasted
- 2 teaspoons extra-virgin olive oil
- 2 teaspoons balsamic vinegar
- ½ teaspoon honey
- Pinch of salt
- Freshly ground pepper to taste

Directions

- Combine greens, figs, goat cheese and almonds in a medium bowl. Stir together oil, vinegar, honey, salt and pepper.
- Just before serving, drizzle the dressing over the salad and toss.

White Bean & Veggie Salad

Ingredients

- 2 cups mixed salad greens
- ¾ cup veggies of your choice, such as chopped cucumbers and cherry tomatoes
- ⅓ cup canned white beans, rinsed and drained
- ½ avocado, diced
- 1 tablespoon red-wine vinegar
- 2 teaspoons extra-virgin olive oil
- ¼ teaspoon kosher salt
- Freshly ground pepper to taste

Directions

- Combine greens, veggies, beans and avocado in a medium bowl. Drizzle with vinegar and oil and season with salt and pepper. Toss to combine and transfer to a large plate.

Greek-Style Chicken Salad

Ingredients

- 2 cups Shredded Chicken Master Recipe
- ½ cup bottled reduced-calorie Greek vinaigrette salad dressing, divided
- 1 teaspoon finely shredded lemon zest
- ½ teaspoon dried oregano, crushed
- 6 cups torn romaine lettuce
- 1 ½ cups chopped cucumber (1 medium)
- 1 cup grape tomatoes, halved
- ¾ cup chopped yellow sweet pepper (1 medium)
- ½ cup thinly sliced red onion, rings separated
- ½ cup crumbled reduced-fat feta cheese (2 ounces)
- ¼ cup pitted Kalamata olives, halved
- 4 Lemon wedges for garnish

Directions

- In a medium bowl, combine chicken, 1/4 cup vinaigrette, lemon zest and oregano; set aside.
- Meanwhile, in a large salad bowl, toss lettuce with the remaining 1/4 cup vinaigrette. Spoon 1 1/2 cups lettuce into each of four shallow bowls. Top each with about 1/3 cup cucumber, 1/4 cup tomatoes, 3 tablespoons sweet pepper, and 2 tablespoons onion. Add chicken mixture to the center of each. Sprinkle with 2 tablespoons feta and 1 tablespoon olives. If desired, serve with lemon wedges.

Quinoa Chickpea Salad with Roasted Red Pepper Hummus Dressing

Ingredients

- 2 tablespoons hummus, original or roasted red pepper flavor
- 1 tablespoon lemon juice
- 1 tablespoon chopped roasted red pepper
- 2 cups mixed salad greens
- ½ cup cooked quinoa
- ½ cup chickpeas, rinsed
- 1 tablespoon unsalted sunflower seeds
- 1 tablespoon chopped fresh parsley
- Pinch of salt
- Pinch of ground pepper

Directions

- Stir hummus, lemon juice and red peppers in a small dish. Thin with water to desired consistency for dressing.
- Arrange greens, quinoa and chickpeas in a large bowl. Top with sunflower seeds, parsley, salt and pepper. Serve with the dressing.

Meal-Prep Falafel Bowls with Tahini Sauce

Ingredients

- 1 (8 ounce) package frozen prepared falafel
- ⅔ cup water
- ½ cup whole-wheat couscous
- 1 (16 ounce) bag steam-in-bag fresh green beans
- 1/2 cup Tahini Sauce (see associated recipe)
- ¼ cup pitted Kalamata olives
- ¼ cup crumbled feta cheese

Directions

- Prepare falafel according to package directions; set aside to cool.
- Bring water to a boil in a small saucepan. Stir in couscous, cover and remove from heat. Allow to stand until the liquid is absorbed, about 5 minutes. Fluff with a fork; set aside.
- Prepare green beans according to package directions.
- Prepare Tahini Sauce. Divide among 4 small condiment containers with lids and refrigerate.
- Divide the green beans among 4 single-serving containers with lids. Top each with 1/2 cup couscous, one-fourth of the falafel and 1 tablespoon each olives and feta. Seal and refrigerate for up to 4 days.
- To serve, reheat in the microwave until heated through, about 2 minutes. Dress with tahini sauce just before eating.

Shrimp, Avocado & Feta Wrap

Ingredients

- 3 ounces chopped cooked shrimp
- ¼ cup diced avocado
- ¼ cup diced tomato
- 1 scallion, sliced
- 2 tablespoons crumbled feta cheese
- 1 tablespoon lime juice
- 1 whole-wheat tortilla

Directions

- Combine shrimp, avocado, tomato, scallion, feta and lime juice in a small bowl. Serve in tortilla.

MEDITERRANEAN SALAD RECIPES

GREEK VILLAGE SALAD

Serves 4

- 4 medium-size ripe tomatoes, cut into wedges
- 1/2 English cucumber, halved and sliced into 1/2-inch slices
- 1 medium cubanelle (green) pepper, stemmed, seeded, halved, and cut into slices
- 1 small red onion, peeled, halved, and thinly sliced
- 1/8 teaspoon salt 1/3 cup extra-virgin olive oil
- 1 1/2 cups cubed feta cheese
- 1 teaspoon dried oregano
- 8 kalamata olives

Directions

- On a serving plate, arrange tomatoes and cucumbers. Next add peppers and onions. Season vegetables with salt.
- Drizzle oil over the vegetables. Top with feta and sprinkle with oregano.
- Finally, top the salad with the olives and serve at room temperature.

STRAWBERRY AND FETA SALAD WITH BALSAMIC DRESSING

Serves 4

- 1 teaspoon Dijon mustard
- 3 tablespoons balsamic vinegar
- 1 clove garlic, peeled and minced
- 3⁄4 cup extra-virgin olive oil
- 1⁄2 teaspoon salt
- 1⁄8 teaspoon pepper
- 4 cups salad greens, rinsed and dried
- 1 pint ripe strawberries, hulled and halved
- 1 1⁄2 cups crumbled feta cheese

Directions

- In a small bowl, whisk the mustard, vinegar, garlic, oil, salt, and pepper to make the dressing.
- In a large bowl, combine the salad greens and the dressing. Plate the salad on a serving platter and top with the strawberries and feta.
- Drizzle any remaining dressing over the salad and serve.

CREAMY CAESAR SALAD

This recipe makes more dressing than you'll need for this salad. Add as much or as little dressing as you prefer. Leftover dressing can be stored in the refrigerator for up to one week.

Serves 6

- 2 cloves garlic, peeled and chopped
- 3 egg yolks
- 1 tablespoon Dijon mustard
- 3 tablespoons Worcestershire sauce
- 1 tablespoon anchovy paste or 2 anchovy fillets
- 1/2 cup grated Parmesan cheese, divided 2 tablespoons fresh lemon juice, divided
- 1/2 teaspoon salt 1 teaspoon pepper
- 1 tablespoon water
- 1 cup light olive oil
- 1 head romaine lettuce, washed, dried, and chopped 1/2 cup chopped cooked bacon 1 cup croutons

Directions

- Place the garlic, egg yolks, mustard, Worcestershire sauce, anchovy paste, 1/4 cup Parmesan cheese, 1 tablespoon lemon juice, salt, pepper, and water into the food processor. Process until the dressing is combined and thick. With the processor running, slowly add the oil until it is well incorporated. Taste the dressing and adjust the seasoning with more salt and pepper, if necessary.

- In a large bowl, combine the lettuce and the remaining lemon juice. Add just enough dressing to coat the lettuce (add more if you want to make it creamier). Toss in the bacon and croutons. Top the salad with the remaining Parmesan. Serve with extra dressing.

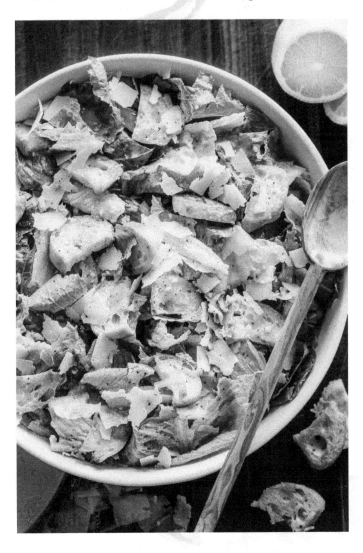

MEDITERRANEAN POULTRY RECIPES

CHIANTI CHICKEN

Serves 4

- 3 cloves garlic, peeled and minced
- 2 tablespoons finely chopped lemon verbena or lemon thyme 2 tablespoons finely chopped fresh parsley
- 2¼ teaspoons salt, divided ⅓ cup and 2 tablespoons extra-virgin olive oil, divided 4 chicken quarters (legs and thighs), rinsed and dried ¾ teaspoon pepper 4 tablespoons unsalted butter, divided
- 2 cups red grapes (in clusters)
- 1 medium red onion, peeled and sliced
- 1 cup Chianti red wine
- 1 cup Chicken or Turkey Stock or Basic Vegetable Stock (see recipes in Chapter 2)

Directions

- Preheat the oven to 400°F. In a small bowl, whisk the garlic, lemon verbena, parsley, ¼ teaspoon of salt, and 2 tablespoons of oil.
- Season the chicken with the remaining salt and pepper. Place your finger between the skin and meat of the chicken thigh and loosen it by moving your finger back and forth to create a pocket. Spread one quarter of the garlic-herb mixture into the pocket. Repeat the process with the remaining chicken quarters.
- Heat the remaining oil and 2 tablespoons of butter in a large oven-safe pot over medium-high heat for 30

seconds. Add the chicken quarters and brown them for 3–4 minutes per side.

- Top the chicken with the grapes. Roast the chicken on the middle rack of the oven for 20–30 minutes or until the chicken's internal temperature reaches 180°F. Remove the chicken and grapes from the pot and keep them warm. Remove any excess fat from the pot.

- Return the pot to the stovetop over medium heat; add the onions and cook for 3–4 minutes. Add the wine and stock, and increase the heat to medium-high. Bring the mixture to a boil, and then reduce the heat to medium-low. Cook the sauce until it thickens. Take the pot off the heat and stir in the remaining butter.

- To serve, put some of the sauce on the bottom of a plate and top with the chicken and grapes. Serve this dish with extra sauce on the side.

CHICKEN BREASTS WITH SPINACH AND FETA

Serves 4

- 1⁄2 cup frozen spinach, thawed, excess water squeezed out 4 tablespoons chopped fresh chives
- 4 tablespoons chopped fresh dill
- 1⁄2 cup crumbled feta cheese
- 1⁄3 cup ricotta cheese
- 4 boneless, skinless chicken breasts
- 11⁄2 teaspoons salt
- 1⁄2 teaspoon pepper
- 1⁄2 teaspoon sweet paprika
- 2 tablespoons extra-virgin olive oil
- 2 tablespoons unsalted butter
- 1⁄2 cup dry white wine
- 2 tablespoons minced red onions
- 1 clove garlic, peeled and smashed
- 2 tablespoons all-purpose flour
- 1 cup Chicken or Turkey Stock
- 1⁄3 cup heavy cream

Directions

- In a medium bowl, combine the spinach, chives, dill, feta, and ricotta. Reserve.
- Using a sharp knife, cut a 3-inch slit into the middle of the thickest part of the chicken breast. The slit should penetrate two-thirds of the way into the chicken breast to

create a pocket. Stuff one-quarter of the spinach-cheese filling into the pocket. Secure the opening with toothpicks. Repeat with the remaining chicken. Then season the chicken with salt, pepper, and paprika.

- Heat the oil and butter in a large skillet over medium-high heat for 30 seconds. Brown the chicken for 3–4 minutes per side. Set the chicken aside and keep it warm. Add the wine to the skillet, and deglaze the pan. Cook for 2 minutes, or until most of the wine has evaporated. Reduce the heat to medium, and stir in the onions, garlic, and flour. Cook for 2 minutes.

- Add the stock, increase the heat to medium-high, and bring the sauce to a boil. Reduce the heat to medium and return the chicken to the skillet. Cover the skillet and cook for 25 minutes. Remove the chicken again and keep it warm. Add the cream and cook until the sauce thickens. Adjust the seasoning with more salt and pepper, if necessary.

- Slice the chicken and put it on the plates. Pour the sauce over the chicken and serve the extra sauce on the side.

CHICKEN TAGINE WITH PRESERVED LEMONS AND OLIVES

Serves 4

- 3 cloves garlic, chopped
- 1 tablespoon chopped fresh ginger
- 1½ preserved lemons, divided 4 medium onions (2 peeled and chopped, 2 peeled and sliced), divided 1 small chili pepper
- 1 tablespoon sweet paprika
- ½ teaspoon ground cumin 2 teaspoons salt, divided
- 2 tablespoons plus 1 cup chopped fresh cilantro
- 2 tablespoons chopped fresh parsley
- ¼ teaspoon saffron threads, soaked in ½ cup hot water
- ½ cup extra-virgin olive oil
- 3 bay leaves
- 4 chicken quarters (legs and thighs), rinsed and dried 2 ripe tomatoes (1 chopped and 1 sliced), divided 2 large potatoes, peeled and cut into wedges
- 1 cup water
- ½ cup pitted green olives

Directions

- To a food processor, add the garlic, ginger, ½ preserved lemon, chopped onions, chili, paprika, cumin, 1 teaspoon salt, 2 tablespoons cilantro, parsley, saffron soaked in water, oil, and bay leaves. Process until everything is chopped and well incorporated. Set the marinade aside.

37

- In a large bowl, combine the chicken and half of the marinade. Toss the chicken to coat it well in the marinade. Season the chicken with the remaining salt.
- In the tagine base (or Dutch oven), put the chopped tomatoes, potatoes, sliced onions, and remaining marinade. Toss to combine and coat the vegetables in the marinade. Add the water to the vegetables and stir. Place the chicken on top of the vegetables. Top the chicken with the tomato slices. Sprinkle with the olives and 1 cup cilantro. Cut the remaining lemon into six wedges and arrange them in the tagine.
- Cover the tagine and place it on the stove over medium-low heat. Cook for 45–50 minutes. Do not stir or uncover the tagine while it is cooking.
- Remove the bay leaves; serve the dish in the tagine at the table.

POMEGRANATE-GLAZED CHICKEN

Serves 4

- 4 bone-in skinless chicken breasts, rinsed and dried 1 teaspoon salt
- 1⁄2 teaspoon pepper
- 2 cups pomegranate juice
- 1⁄8 teaspoon ground mastiha
- 2 teaspoons grated orange zest
- 3 cloves garlic, peeled and smashed
- 1 teaspoon dried rosemary

Directions

- Preheat the oven to 375°F. Season the chicken with the salt and pepper. Place the chicken on a baking sheet lined with parchment paper. Bake the chicken on the middle rack in the oven for 25–30 minutes or until the chicken's internal temperature is 180°F.
- In a small pan over medium-high heat, combine the pomegranate juice, mastiha, orange zest, garlic, and rosemary. Bring the mixture to a boil, reduce the heat to medium-low, and cook until the sauce reduces to 1⁄4 cup and has a syrup-like consistency. Remove the garlic and take the sauce off the heat.
- Brush the chicken with the reserved sauce and serve the remaining sauce on the side.

MEDITERRANEAN SEAFOOD RECIPES

RED MULLET SAVORO STYLE

Serves 4

- 4 (1⁄2-pound) whole red mullet, cleaned, gutted, and scaled 2 teaspoons salt
- 1 cup all-purpose flour
- 2⁄3 cup extra-virgin olive oil, divided 6 or 7 sprigs fresh rosemary
- 8 cloves garlic, peeled and coarsely chopped
- 2⁄3 cup red wine vinegar

Directions

- Rinse the fish and pat them dry with a paper towel. Season both sides and the cavity of the fish with salt. Let them sit for 20 minutes. Dredge the fish in flour and set aside.
- Heat 1⁄3 cup of oil in a frying pan over medium-high heat for 1 minute or until the oil is hot. Fry the fish (in batches) for 4–5 minutes a side or until golden. Place the fish on a serving platter. Discard the frying oil and wipe the pan clean.
- Add the remaining oil to the pan and heat for 1 minute. Add the rosemary; fry until it crisps and turns an olive color. Remove the rosemary from the oil. Stir the garlic into the oil and keep stirring until the garlic turns golden. Immediately add the vinegar. Stir until the sauce has thickened and becomes a little sweet.
- Pour the sauce over the fish and serve immediately. Garnish the fish with the fried rosemary.

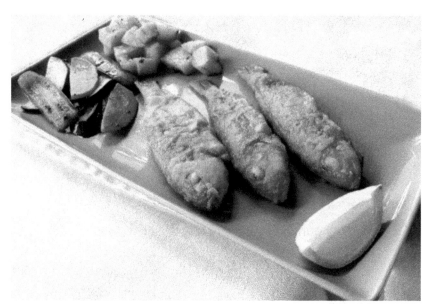

SPINACH-STUFFED SOLE

Serves 4

- 1⁄4 cup extra-virgin olive oil, divided 4 scallions, ends trimmed and sliced
- 1 pound package frozen spinach, thawed and drained
- 3 tablespoons chopped fennel fronds, or tarragon
- 1 teaspoon salt, divided
- 1⁄2 teaspoon pepper, divided 4 (6-ounce) sole fillets, skins removed
- 2 tablespoons plus
- 11⁄2 teaspoons grated lemon zest, divided
- 1 teaspoon sweet paprika

Directions

- Preheat the oven to 400°F. Heat 2 tablespoons of oil in a medium skillet over medium heat for 30 seconds. Add the scallions and cook them for 3–4 minutes. Allow the scallions to cool to room temperature.
- In a bowl, combine the scallions, spinach, and fennel. Season the ingredients with 1⁄2 teaspoon of salt and 1⁄4 teaspoon of pepper.
- Rinse the fish fillets and pat them dry with a paper towel. Rub the fish with the remaining oil and sprinkle them with 2 tablespoons of lemon zest. Season the fillets with remaining salt and pepper, and sprinkle them with the paprika.

- Divide the spinach filling among the fillets; to ensure that the fillets don't unravel when baking, place the stuffing on the skin side. Roll up each fillet, starting from the widest end. Use two toothpicks to secure each fillet. Place the fillets on a baking sheet lined with parchment paper, and drizzle the remaining oil over them.
- Bake on the middle rack of the oven for 15–20 minutes. Remove the toothpicks and sprinkle the fillets with the remaining lemon zest. Serve immediately.

GRILLED OCTOPUS

Serves 4

- 2 1/2- to 3-pound octopus, cleaned and beak removed 3 bay leaves
- 1/4 cup red wine 3 tablespoons balsamic vinegar, divided
- 2/3 cup extra-virgin olive oil, divided 1 teaspoon dried oregano
- 1 teaspoon salt
- 1 teaspoon pepper
- 1 large lemon, cut into wedges

Directions

- Put the octopus and bay leaves in a large pot over medium-high heat. Cover the pot and cook the octopus for 5–8 minutes. Uncover the pot to see whether the octopus has released some liquid (about a cup). If the octopus hasn't released its liquid, just cover and continue cooking for another 5 minutes or until it has released its liquid. Reduce the heat to medium-low and cook for 45 minutes or until the octopus is tender.
- Add the wine and 2 tablespoons of vinegar. Remove the pot from the heat and allow the octopus to cool to room temperature in the liquid.
- Preheat a gas or charcoal grill to medium-high. Remove the octopus from the liquid and cut it into pieces, leaving each tentacle whole. In a large bowl, combine the octopus,

1/3 cup of oil, the oregano, and the remaining vinegar. Season it with the salt and pepper.

- Place the octopus on the grill and cook for 2–3 minutes a side.
- Drizzle the grilled octopus with the remaining oil and serve it with the lemon wedges.

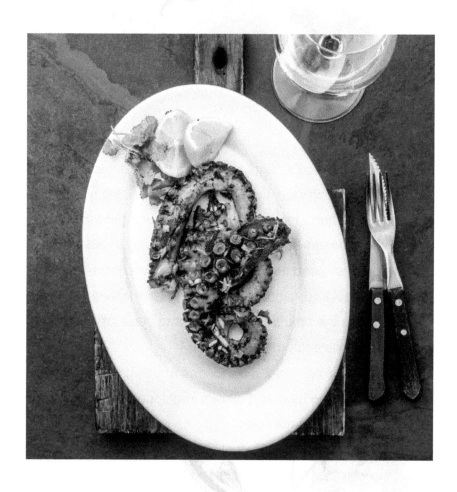

SCALLOPS SAGANAKI

Serves 4

- 16 medium scallops, rinsed and patted dry
- 1 teaspoon salt
- 1/2 teaspoon pepper 1/2 cup extra-virgin olive oil 1/3 cup dry white wine
- 2 ounces ouzo
- 2 tablespoons fresh lemon juice
- 6 cloves garlic, peeled and thinly sliced
- 1 small red chili pepper, stemmed and thinly sliced
- 1/2 teaspoon sweet paprika 1 small leek, ends trimmed, thoroughly cleaned, cut lengthwise, and julienned into matchsticks 2/3 cup bread crumbs 2 tablespoons chopped fresh parsley
- 1 large lemon, cut into wedges

Directions

- Preheat the oven to 450°F. Season both sides of the scallops with the salt and pepper. Place the scallops in a medium baking dish (or divide them among four small baking dishes or ramekins). Set aside.
- In a medium bowl, whisk the oil, wine, ouzo, lemon juice, garlic, chili, and sweet paprika. Pour the sauce over the scallops; top with the leeks and then the bread crumbs.
- Bake on the middle rack for 8–10 minutes. Set the oven to broil and bake for another 2–3 minutes or until the bread crumbs are golden.

- Let the scallops cool for 5 minutes and top them with parsley. Serve the scallops with the lemon wedges.

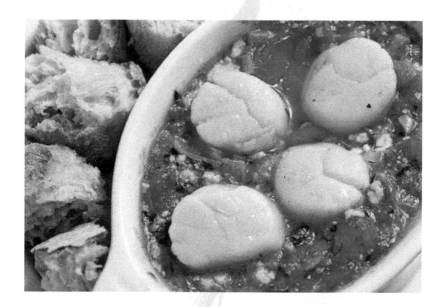

MEDITERRANEAN MEAT, BEEF AND PORK RECIPES

PORK CHOPS IN WINE

Serves 4

4 thick-cut pork chops

1/2 cup extra-virgin olive oil

1 cup white wine

1/2 cup hot water

1 tablespoon dried oregano Salt and pepper to taste

Directions

- Rinse pork chops well and pat dry with a paper towel.
- Place 2 tablespoons olive oil in a frying pan; lightly brown pork chops.
- Put remaining olive oil in a fresh pan and turn heat to medium-high. Cook pork chops 3–4 minutes per side, making sure to turn them over at least once.
- Add wine; bring to a boil. Turn to medium and simmer for 10 minutes, turning the meat once.
- Add 1/2 cup hot water to pan; bring to a boil and let simmer until the sauce has reduced. Sprinkle with oregano, salt, and pepper, and serve immediately.

BREADED PORK CHOPS

Serves 6

- 3 slices raisin-pumpernickel bread
- 6 cloves garlic
- 1/2 cup applesauce 1 teaspoon olive oil
- 6 pork chops
- Fresh-cracked black pepper, to taste
- Kosher salt, to taste

Directions

- Preheat oven to 375°F. Spray a baking sheet with cooking spray.
- Toast the bread and grate into crumbs. Mince the garlic in a blender, then add the applesauce and oil, and blend until smooth.
- Rub the chops with the garlic-applesauce mixture. Bread with pumpernickel crumbs and place on prepared baking sheet. Spray the chops with cooking spray and season with pepper and salt.
- Bake for 20 minutes, then turn and bake for 20–40 minutes longer, depending on the thickness of the pork. Serve hot.

SMYRNA SOUTZOUKAKIA

Serves 4

- 2 slices white bread
- 1/2 cup white wine, divided
- 1 pound lean ground beef
- 2 medium onions, peeled (1 grated, 1 diced), divided 4 cloves garlic, minced, divided
- 3 tablespoons finely chopped fresh parsley
- 1/2 teaspoon plus 1/8 teaspoon ground cumin, divided 1 teaspoon dried oregano
- 2 1/2 teaspoons salt, divided 3/4 teaspoon pepper, divided 1 large egg, beaten
- 1/2 cup extra-virgin olive oil, divided
- 1 bay leaf
- 1 (28-ounce) can plum tomatoes, puréed
- 1/8 teaspoon cinnamon

Directions

- Soak the bread in 1/4 cup of the wine, squeeze out the liquid, and crumble the bread. In a large bowl, mix the beef, bread, grated onion, 1 teaspoon of the garlic, parsley, 1/2 teaspoon of the cumin, oregano, 2 teaspoons of the salt, 1/2 teaspoon of the pepper, and the egg. Mix well and refrigerate for 1 hour.

- Heat 1/4 cup of the oil in a medium skillet over medium-high heat for 30 seconds. Add the diced onions, bay leaf, tomatoes, remaining garlic, remaining cumin, cinnamon, and remaining wine. Season with the remaining salt and pepper. Reduce the heat to medium-low and cook for 30 minutes.

- Form the meat mixture into 3-inch, quenelle-shaped sausages. Preheat a gas or charcoal grill to medium-high. Place the sausages on the grill and grill them 3–4 minutes a side (if you prefer to fry them instead, lightly dredge them in flour before frying them in olive oil).
- Place the sausages in the tomato sauce and cook for 10–15 minutes.
- Remove the bay leaf and serve hot.

STUFFED PEPPERS WITH MEAT

Serves 6

- 1⁄3 cup extra-virgin olive oil 2 medium onions, peeled and diced
- 3 cloves garlic, peeled and minced
- 1 cup finely chopped fresh parsley
- 1 cup finely chopped fresh dill
- 2 tablespoons finely chopped fresh mint
- 1 cup tomato sauce
- 1 cup long-grain rice
- 2 pounds lean ground beef
- 21⁄2 teaspoons salt
- 3⁄4 teaspoon pepper 2–3 cups hot water

Directions

- Preheat the oven to 375°F. Heat the oil in a large skillet over medium-high heat for 30 seconds. Reduce the heat to medium, and add the onions and garlic. Cook for 10 minutes or until the onions soften. Add the parsley, dill, mint, and tomato sauce. Cook for 10 minutes or until the sauce thickens. Take the skillet off the heat and cool it for 5 minutes.
- Add the rice and ground beef to the skillet. Season with the salt and pepper and cook until rice is soft and beef is browned.
- Spoon the beef-rice mixture into the peppers and place them in a roasting pan that will hold all the peppers snugly.

Add 2–3 cups of hot water, enough to fill the pan up to 1 inch on the sides of the peppers.

- Bake on the middle rack of the oven for 70–80 minutes or until the pepper tops are golden and the rice is cooked.
- Serve hot or at room temperature.

VEGETARIAN AND LEGUMES MEDITERRANEAN RECIPES

ITALIAN GREEN BEANS WITH POTATOES

Serves 6

- 1 tablespoon extra-virgin olive oil
- 1 1/4 pounds Italian green beans, trimmed 2 cloves garlic, peeled and minced
- 2 large potatoes, peeled, cooked, and diced
- 1/2 cup Basic Vegetable Stock
- 1/2 teaspoon dried oregano
- 1/4 cup chopped fresh parsley
- 1 teaspoon salt
- 1/2 teaspoon pepper
- 1/4 cup chopped walnuts, toasted

Directions

- Heat the oil in a large skillet over medium heat for 30 seconds.
- Add the beans, garlic, potatoes, stock, oregano, parsley, salt, and pepper. Cook for 8–10 minutes or until the beans are tender.
- Adjust the seasoning with more salt and pepper, if necessary. Sprinkle the walnuts over the beans and serve.

ZUCCHINI PIE WITH HERBS AND CHEESE

Serves 12

- 1⁄2 cup extra-virgin olive oil 12 scallions, ends trimmed and finely chopped
- 4 medium zucchini, 3 diced and 1 thinly sliced into rounds
- 1⁄2 teaspoon salt
- 5 large eggs
- 1 cup self-rising flour
- 1 teaspoon baking powder
- 1 cup strained Greek yogurt
- 1 cup crumbled feta cheese
- 1 cup grated kasseri (or Gouda) cheese
- 1 teaspoon pepper
- 2 teaspoons sweet paprika, divided
- 1 cup chopped fresh dill

Directions

- Preheat the oven to 350°F. Heat the oil in a large skillet over medium heat for 30 seconds. Add the scallions, diced zucchini, and salt. Cook for about 20 minutes to soften the vegetables and evaporate half of their released liquids. Take the skillet off the heat and reserve.
- Crack the eggs into a large bowl and whisk for 2 minutes. Stir in the flour and baking powder. Stir in the Greek yogurt. Stir in the cheeses and softened vegetables. Stir in the pepper, 1 1⁄2 teaspoons of paprika, and the dill.

- Pour the mixture into a large, deep, greased baking dish. Top the vegetables with zucchini slices and sprinkle with the remaining paprika.
- Place the dish on the middle rack and bake for 1 hour. Allow the pie to cool for about 15 minutes before cutting it into slices and serving.

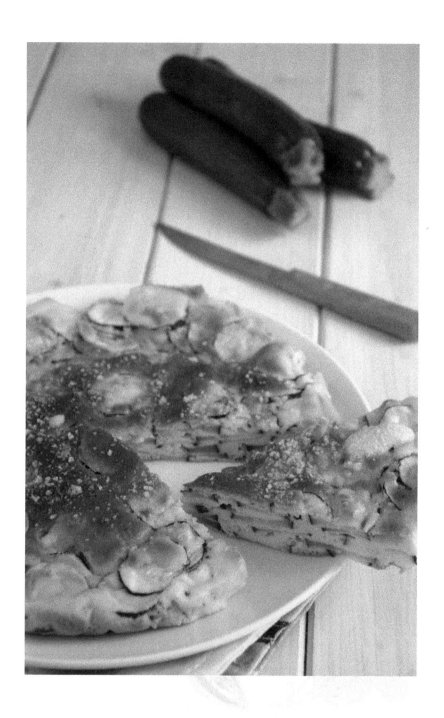

POTATO AND FENNEL GRATIN

Serves 10

- 1 tablespoon unsalted butter, softened
- 1⁄4 cup extra-virgin olive oil
- 4 cups sliced fennel, trimmed and outer layer removed
- 1 large onion, peeled and sliced
- 4 or 5 large Yukon gold potatoes, peeled and thinly sliced
- 1 cup heavy cream
- 1 cup whole milk
- 1 tablespoon fresh thyme leaves
- 1 teaspoon salt, divided
- 1⁄2 teaspoon pepper, divided
- 21⁄2 cups grated Gouda cheese, divided
- 1⁄2 cup bread crumbs

Directions

- Preheat the oven to 375°F. Grease a large, deep baking dish with the butter.
- Heat the oil in a large skillet over medium heat for 30 seconds. Add the fennel and onions. Cook the vegetables for 15 minutes or until they are soft and translucent. Set aside.
- In a large bowl, combine the potatoes, cream, milk, and thyme. Layer the bottom of the baking dish with one-third of the potato slices (leave cream/milk in bowl for later). Spread half of the fennel mixture evenly over the potatoes. Sprinkle 1⁄2 teaspoon of the salt and 1⁄4

teaspoon of the pepper over the fennel mixture and top with 1 cup of the cheese. Repeat another potato layer, another fennel and cheese layer, and finish with a final layer of potatoes.

- Pour enough of the cream/milk over the baking dish to just cover the gratin. Using your fingers, press down gently to even out and compact the potatoes. Sprinkle the remaining cheese evenly over the top. Sprinkle the bread crumbs over the top.

- Bake the gratin for 90 minutes or until the potatoes are very tender and the top is brown and bubbling. Allow the gratin to cool for 20 minutes before slicing and serving.

EGGPLANT ROLL-UPS

Serves 6

- 5 ounces ricotta cheese
- 5 ounces feta cheese, crumbled
- 1 large egg
- 1/2 cup pine nuts, toasted 3 tablespoons bread crumbs
- 1 tablespoon chopped fresh mint
- 1 tablespoon chopped fresh dill
- 1 teaspoon salt, divided
- 1 teaspoon pepper, divided
- 1/4 cup plus 2 tablespoons extra-virgin olive oil, divided 1 medium onion, peeled and chopped
- 3 cloves garlic, peeled and minced
- 1 (28-ounce) can whole plum tomatoes, hand crushed
- 1 tablespoon chopped fresh parsley
- 1 teaspoon dried oregano
- 4 long, slender Japanese eggplants
- 16 medium slices mozzarella cheese

Directions

- In a large bowl combine ricotta, feta, egg, pine nuts, bread crumbs, mint, dill, 1/4 teaspoon salt, and 1/4 teaspoon pepper. Set aside.
- Heat 1/4 cup oil in a large skillet over medium heat. Add the onions and garlic, and cook for 5–7 minutes or until softened. Stir in tomatoes and bring to a boil. Reduce the heat to medium and simmer for 10 minutes until the

sauce thickens. Stir in the parsley, oregano, 1/4 teaspoon salt, and 1/4 teaspoon pepper. Remove the sauce from the heat and set it aside.

- Set the oven to broil. Cut the eggplants lengthwise into 16 (1/4-inch) slices. Brush both sides of the slices with the remaining oil and season them with the remaining salt and pepper. Place the slices on a baking sheet, and broil them on one side for 3 minutes. Allow the eggplant to cool slightly. Preheat the oven to 350°F.

- Spread half of the tomato sauce on the bottom of a large casserole dish. Spread 2 tablespoons of the cheese filling on the surface of each eggplant slice, and roll it up to form a bundle. Place the eggplant roll-up in the dish (seam-side down) on top of the tomato sauce. Repeat with the remaining eggplant slices. Pour the remaining tomato sauce over the roll-ups.

- Top each roll-up with a slice of mozzarella cheese. Bake for 30–45 minutes or until the mozzarella is brown and bubbling. Serve immediately.

MEDITERRANEAN DESSERTS

ALMOND TANGERINE BITES

Yields approximately 20–25 pieces

- 2 cups raw almonds
- 5 tangerines
- 1 cup brown sugar
- Icing sugar

Directions

- Blanch almonds by boiling them in water; when they start floating to the top they can be removed from the water, drained, and easily peeled. Boil 3 tangerines in a generous amount of water for 5 minutes to remove the bitterness from the rind.
- Squeeze juice from remaining 2 tangerines and set aside; discard skins.
- Peel 3 boiled tangerines and put skins along with blanched almonds into a blender; purée until very finely ground.
- Remove puréed almond mix from blender; in large bowl, mix with brown sugar.
- Slowly add tangerine juice while continuing to mix well.
- Roll small pieces of mixture into walnut-size balls using the palms of your hands; set aside on a sheet of wax paper to dry.
- Dust balls lightly with icing sugar before serving.

AMYGDALOTA (ALMOND BISCUITS)

Yields approximately 25–30 pieces

- 1 pound blanched almonds
- 1 tablespoon fine semolina
- 3 eggs, separated
- 1½ cups sugar
- 1 tablespoon orange blossom water

Directions

- Preheat the oven to 350°F.
- Purée blanched almonds and semolina in a food processor until very fine.
- Beat 2 egg yolks and 1 egg white well with a mixer in a large bowl; add sugar, almond purée, and orange blossom water. Mix well with a dough hook (stand mixer) or a wooden spoon.
- In a mixing bowl, whip 2 egg whites until nice and stiff with peaks; incorporate thoroughly into the almond purée mixture.
- Take up small pieces of dough and roll into balls between your palms. Place balls on a cookie sheet and press an almond into the center of each, flattening lower hemisphere of biscuit.
- Bake for 20–30 minutes, or until cookies are starting to turn slightly golden. Remove from the oven and leave to cool for at least 1 hour. Important: To maintain the inner chewiness of these biscuits, it is a good idea to store them

in sealed, airtight containers or wrapped in cellophane/plastic.

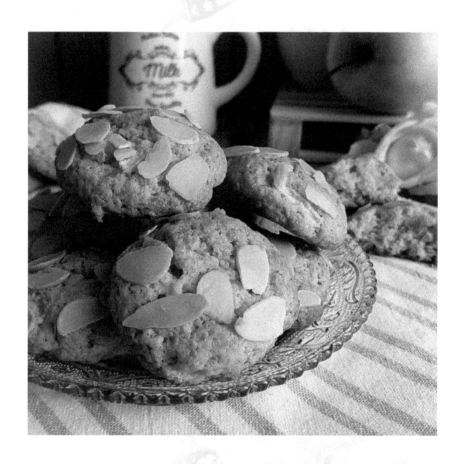

CYPRIOT LOUKOUMIA

Yields approximately 20 pieces

- 1⁄2 cup butter 2 cups flour
- 11⁄2 cups milk
- 1⁄2 cup sugar
- 1 egg, beaten
- 1 teaspoon baking powder
- 1⁄2 cup orange marmalade
- 1 cup finely chopped almonds
- 2 tablespoons orange blossom water
- 1⁄2 teaspoon cinnamon
- 1⁄2 teaspoon nutmeg Confectioners' sugar

Directions

- Preheat the oven to 350°F.
- Melt butter in a pot over medium-high heat. Slowly add flour, stirring constantly with a wooden spoon to avoid clumping.
- Lower heat to medium-low and slowly add milk, making sure to stir continuously as the mixture thickens and starts clumping.
- When all the milk has been added, remove from heat and add sugar, egg, and baking powder; mix well until the dough is uniformly smooth.
- Prepare the filling by mixing the marmalade, almonds, orange blossom water, cinnamon, and nutmeg.

- Using a rolling pin, spread pieces of dough on a floured surface to uniform thickness of a banana peel.
- Place a small amount of filling mixture in the center of each disc. Fold each disc in half over the filling into a half-moon shape; tightly pinch together edges to ensure a good seal.
- Place cookies on a buttered pan and bake for 20 minutes. Let stand for 30 minutes. Sprinkle cookies with confectioners' sugar before serving.

GALATOPITA (MILK PIE)

Serves 6

- 5 cups milk
- 1/2 cup butter 1 cup sugar
- 1 cup fine semolina
- 3 eggs
- Ground cinnamon or icing sugar for sprinkling

Directions

- Preheat the oven to 350°F.
- On the stovetop, bring milk almost to a boil in a saucepan. Add butter, sugar, and semolina, making sure to stir continuously until thick crème is formed. Turn off the heat and let stand a couple of minutes to cool slightly.
- Beat eggs and add to thickened mixture; whisk well.
- Butter or oil the sides and bottom of a pie dish or other high-walled oven pan. Pour in mixture; bake for approximately 1 hour, until the top has browned. Turn off the oven but do not remove the pie for another 15 minutes.
- Once the pie is removed from the oven, let it stand for a couple of hours. Serve topped with cinnamon or icing sugar. Can also be topped with fruit preserve or jam of your choosing.

MEDITERRANEAN
BREAD

GARLIC BREAD

Serves 6

- 1 cup extra-virgin olive oil
- 2 cloves garlic, peeled and minced
- 1 sun-dried tomato, minced
- 1⁄4 cup chopped fresh chives
- 2 tablespoons chopped fresh parsley
- 1 teaspoon dried rosemary
- 1 teaspoon dried oregano
- 1 teaspoon salt
- 1⁄4 teaspoon red pepper flakes 1 (20-inch) baguette

Directions

- Preheat the oven to 300°F. In a small bowl, whisk the oil, garlic, tomato, chives, parsley, rosemary, oregano, salt, and red pepper flakes. Continue whisking until the ingredients are well incorporated.
- Slice the baguette lengthwise, but leave the back seam intact. Spread the garlic mixture evenly inside both the top and bottom of the baguette. Let it sink into the bread. Fold the bread closed.
- Wrap the bread in aluminum foil and bake it for 15–20 minutes.
- Unwrap the garlic bread and serve it warm.

RUFFLED-PHYLLO CHEESE PIE

Serves 12

- 3 large eggs
- 1/2 cup whole milk 2 cups crumbled feta cheese
- 2 cups ricotta cheese
- 1/4 teaspoon pepper
- 1/2 cup unsalted butter, melted 1 package phyllo pastry, thawed, at room temperature
- 1 (12-ounce) can club soda or sparkling water

Directions

- Preheat the oven to 375°F. In a large bowl, whisk the eggs and milk. Stir in the feta, ricotta, and pepper. Mix well, breaking up the large pieces of feta with your spoon. Reserve the filling.
- Brush butter on the bottom of a 13" × 9" baking pan. Open the package of phyllo and lay the sheets flat on a work surface. Cover the sheets with a slightly damp tea towel. Phyllo dries quickly so keep the sheets covered.
- Place a sheet of phyllo on a work surface. Spread 3 tablespoons of the cheese filling over the sheet. Loosely fold about 1 inch of phyllo from the bottom over the filling and lightly pinch the right and left ends. Continue to loosely fold, over and under so it looks like ruffled curtains, and lightly pinch the ends together. Set the folded phyllo sheet in the baking pan with the ruffles facing up, not lying down. Repeat with the remaining

- phyllo sheets, and set them in the pan leaning against each other until the pan is full.
- Brush the tops of the phyllo with butter. Pour the club soda or sparkling water over the entire surface. Bake the pie on the middle rack of the oven for 35–45 minutes or until it turns golden brown.
- Remove the pie from the oven and allow it to cool for 5–10 minutes. Cut the pie into squares and serve.

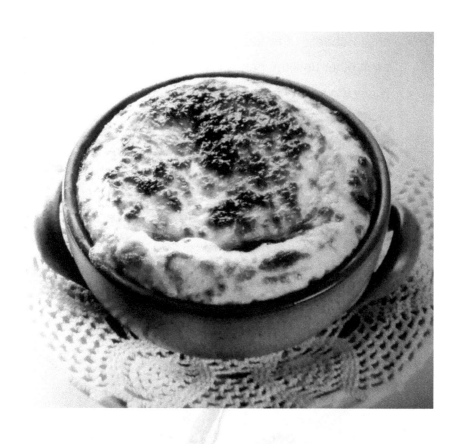

MEDITERRANEAN
RICE AND GRAINS

Japanese Onigiri Rice Triangles Recipe

Mediterranean version

Ingredients

- 1½ cups uncooked short grain white rice
- 1 2/3 cups water
- ½ teaspoon salt
- ½ ounce dried sliced seaweed, finely chopped (2 tablespoons)
- 1 tablespoon sesame seeds
- 4 ounces cooked, smoked, or canned salmon
- 1 sheet nori

Preparation

- Measure the rice in a medium saucepan. Rinse, stir, and drain it several times. Cover it with plenty of water and allow it to soak for about 40 minutes or until the rice is an opaque white color. Thoroughly drain the rice in a mesh strainer.
- Return the drained rice to the saucepan. Add water and salt; cover the pot. Bring it to a boil over high heat, then reduce heat to maintain a simmer. Cook the rice for 20 minutes, then remove it from the heat. Leave the pot covered and allow the rice to steam for another 10 minutes to finish the cooking process.
- Sprinkle in the seaweed and sesame seeds. Stir to combine.

- When the rice mixture is cool enough to handle, moisten both hands. Spread about ½ cup of the rice out on the palm of one hand. Place 1 tablespoon of salmon in the center, and form the rice mixture into a ball around it. Press firmly to stick the rice together. Form it into the traditional triangle shape, flat on both sides, with rounded corners.
- Using scissors, cut the sheet of nori into strips, 1 x 2 ½-inches each; wrap a strip of nori around one edge of the triangle. Cover or wrap tightly until serving.

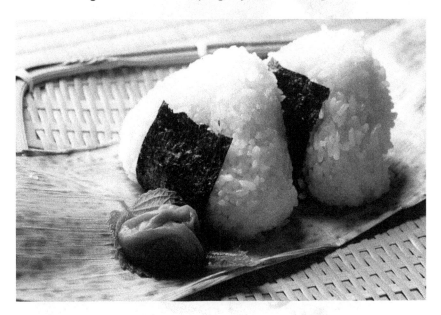

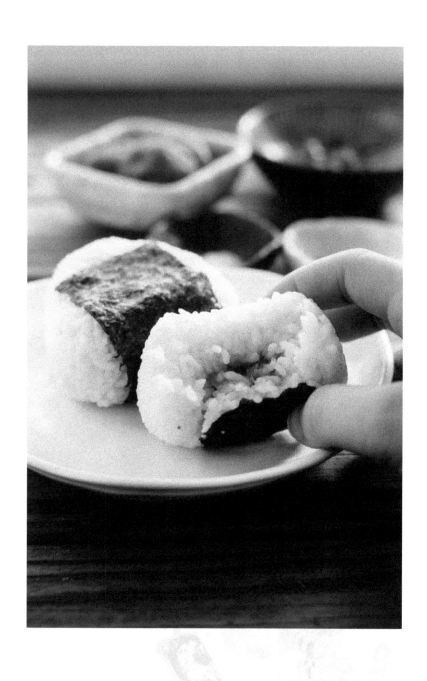

MEDITERRANEAN EGG AND RECIPIES

Mediterranean-Breakfast-Burrito

Ingredients

- 6 tortillas whole 10 inch - I use sun-dried tomato
- 9 eggs whole
- 2 cups baby spinach washed and dried
- 3 tbsp black olives sliced
- 3 tbsp sun-dried tomatoes chopped
- ½ cup feta cheese I use light/low-fat feta
- ¾ cup refried beans canned
- Garnish: salsa (optional)

Instructions

- Spray medium frying pan with non- stick spray. Scramble eggs and toss for about 5 minutes, or until eggs are no longer liquid. Add spinach, black olives, sun-dried tomatoes and continue to stir/toss until no longer wet. Add feta cheese and cover until cheese is melted.
- Add 2 tbsp of refried beans to each tortilla. Top with egg mixture, dividing evenly between all burritos. Wrap as shown in video.
- Grill on panini press (this is what I use but you don't have to have one) or in frying pan until lightly browned.
- Serve hot with salsa and fruit (optional)
- If freezing: wait until cooled, then wrap as directed in video.
- If you are reheating: Heat in microwave (in parchment paper) for about 2 minutes. Serve hot.

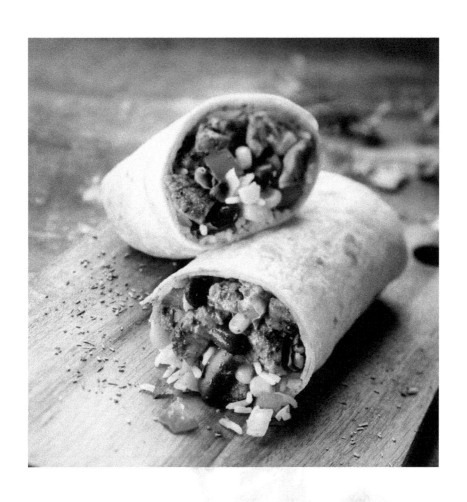

MEDITERRANEAN
BREAKFAST BAKE

Deidre's Low Carb Bread Recipe Using a Bread Machine

Ingredients

- 1 cup warm Water about 90-100°
- 1 TBS Dry Active yeast
- 1 tsp Allulose Liquid form
- 2 Eggs slightly beaten
- ⅔ cup Ground Golden flax meal
- ½ cup Oat Fiber
- 1¼ cup Vital Wheat Gluten
- 4 tbs Allulose Powdered sugar form Use can use the same about of Swerve or Erythritol too
- 1 tbs of psyllium husk powder
- 1 tsp Pink Salt
- 2 tbs softened butter

Instructions

1. Add to the bread machine in this exact order:
2. Add the warm water and yeast and let it sit for 5 to 7 minutes until it foams slightly.
3. Add the liquid Allulose.
4. Add the whipped eggs.
5. Add the ground golden flax meal.
6. Add the oat fiber.
7. Add the vital wheat gluten.
8. Add the powdered allulose sweetener.
9. Add the psyllium husk powder.

10. Add the pink salt

11. Add the room temperature butter.

12. Close the lid of the bread machine and set the machine to mix and bake at 3 hours.

13. Remove the bread from the bread machine pan and allow it to cool before slicing it.

NOTES

2 carbs per slice @ 16 slices per loaf.

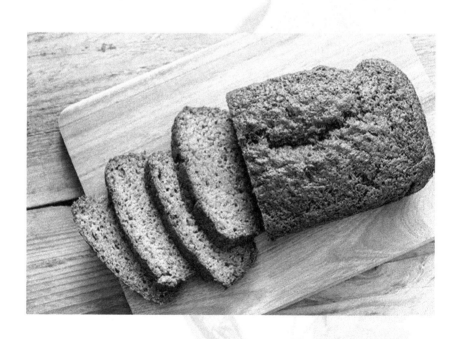

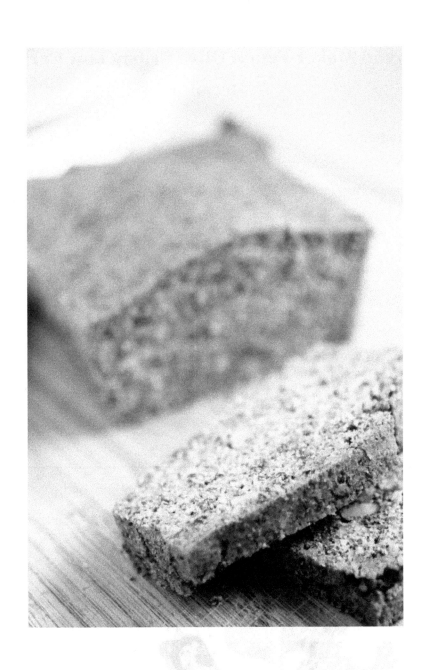

Bread Maker Feta & Olive Crusty Low Carb Bread

Ingredients

- 1 cup warm water
- 2 tbsp inulin or 1 tbsp honey or sugar
- 1 tbsp yeast
- 2 eggs lightly whisked
- 60 g butter cubed
- 2/3 cup chia flour (70g)
- 1/2 cup Macro Gentle Fibre (50g)
- 1 1/4 cups Gluten Flour (170g)
- Pinch salt flakes
- 1/2 tsp xanthan gum

Filling

- 180 g feta cheese cut into 1 cm cubes
- 180 g kalamata olives pitted and roughly chopped
- 1 tbsp fresh parsley finely chopped (optional)

Instructions

1. Remove Bread Pan from Bread Maker. Check that the kneading blade placed in position in the base of the pan.
2. Combine warm water, inulin (or sweetener) and yeast into a small bowl and mix until foamy. Pour into bread pan.
3. Add remaining bread ingredients in ingredients order into bread pan and place back into Bread Maker.
4. Select Menu 3 - White Stuffed Bread and press Start.

5. After about 20-25 minutes you will hear a beeping sound. Add the feta, kalamata olives and parsley to pan and close lid. Press start to continue.

6. When the Bread Maker beeps next it is time to turn it off and remove your bread. Use oven mit as the bread pan will be hot. Turn the bread out of pan. It should pop out easily. Leave to cool on a wire rack completely before slicing.

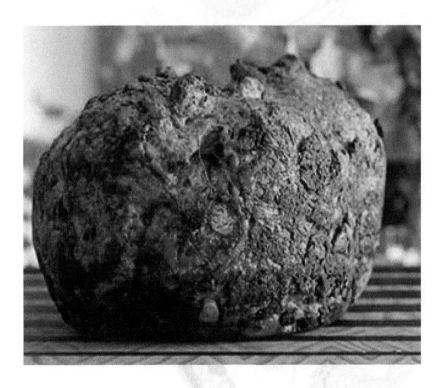

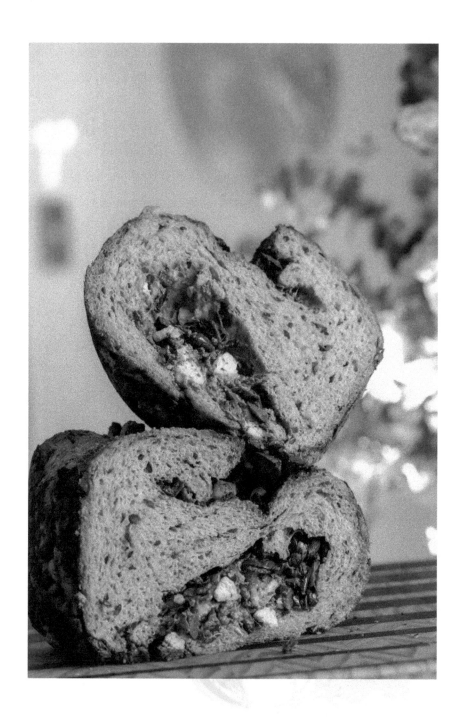

Gluten Free & Keto Bread With Yeast

Ingredients

For The Paleo & Keto Bread

- 2 teaspoons active dry yeast
- 2 teaspoons inulin or maple sirup, honey, to feed the yeast*
- 120 ml water lukewarm between 105-110°F
- 168 g almond flour **
- 83 g golden flaxseed meal finely ground
- 15 g whey protein isolate
- 18 g psyllium husk finely ground
- 2 teaspoons xanthan gum or 4 teaspoons ground flaxseed meal**
- 2 teaspoons baking powder
- 1 teaspoon kosher salt
- 1/4 teaspoon cream of tartar
- 1/8 teaspoon ground ginger
- 1 egg at room temperature
- 110 g egg whites about 3, at room temperature
- 56 g grass-fed unsalted butter or ghee, melted and cooled
- 1 tablespoon apple cider vinegar
- 58 g sour cream or coconut cream + 2 tsp apple cider vinegar

Instructions

For The Paleo & Keto Bread

- Add yeast and maple syrup (to feed the yeast, see notes) to a large bowl. Heat up water to 105-110°F, and if you don't have a thermometer it should only feel lightly warm to touch. Pour water over yeast mixture, cover bowl with a kitchen towel and allow to rest for 7 minutes. The mixture should be bubbly, if it isn't start again (too cold water won't activate the yeast and too hot will kill it).

- Mix your flours while the yeast is proofing. Add almond flour, flaxseed meal, whey protein powder, psyllium husk, xanthan gum, baking powder, salt, cream of tartar and ginger to a medium bowl and whisk until thoroughly mixed. Set aside.

- Once your yeast is proofed, add in the egg, egg whites, lightly cooled melted butter (you don't want to scramble the eggs or kill the yeast!) and vinegar. Mix with an electric mixer for a couple minutes until light and frothy. Add the flour mixture in two batches, alternating with the sour cream, and mixing until thoroughly incorporated. You want to mix thoroughly and quickly to activate the xanthan gum, though the dough will become thick as the flours absorb the moisture.

- Transfer bread dough to prepared loaf pan, using a wet spatula to even out the top. Cover with a kitchen towel and place in a warm draft-free space for 50-60 minutes until the dough has risen just past the top of the loaf pan. How long it takes depends on your altitude, temperature and

92

humidity- so keep an eye out for it every 15 minutes or so. And keep in mind that if you use a larger loaf pan it won't rise past the top.

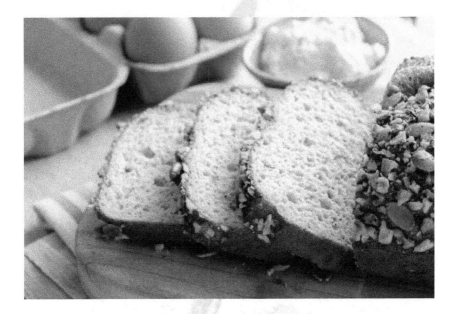

Keto Farmer's Yeast Bread Loaf

Ingredients

- 2 1/4 cup warm (like bath water) water, divided
- 2 teaspoons sugar*
- 2 envelopes (4 1/2 teaspoons) active dry yeast
- 2 cups vital wheat gluten
- 2 cups super fine almond flour
- 1/2 cup flaxseed meal, ground in a blender for 2 minutes
- 1 teaspoon salt
- 3 teaspoons baking powder
- 6 tablespoons olive oil
- 1/2 tablespoon butter, melted

Instructions

1. Liberally grease a 10 inch wide glass or metal bowl with butter.
2. Add a 1/2 cup warm water to another large bowl and mix in sugar until dissolved. Mix in yeast and cover the bowl with a towel. After 7-10 minutes the mixture should be frothy with small bubbles. If it is not frothy, then the yeast is dead and you need to start over with fresh yeast.
3. As you are waiting for the yeast to proof, mix together all dry ingredients in a large bowl. Sift the dry ingredients through a sifter or a sieve.
4. Add remaining 1 3/4 cup water and olive oil to the frothy yeast mixture and stir to combine.

5. Slowly add the dry ingredients to the wet and stir with a wooden spoon until fully combined.

6. The dough should be sticky and rather wet. If it is too dry to knead, then add a little bit more water. Knead the dough for 3 minutes. Do not over knead.

7. Form the dough into a ball and place in the greased bowl.

8. Preheat the oven for 2-3 minutes until the temperature reaches 100-110 degrees. Cover the bowl with a towel and place in the warm oven to rise for 1 hour. Remove from the oven.

9. Preheat the oven to 350 degrees F and melt the butter in a small bowl in the microwave. Brush the butter over the top of the dough.

10. Place the bowl in the oven and bake for 35-45 minutes until the internal temperature reaches 190-200 degrees F. The closer to 200 degrees that you get, the thicker the crust.

11. Cool in the bowl for 10 minutes. Then place a large cutting board over the bowl. Invert the bowl to release the bread.

12. Cool completely before cutting.

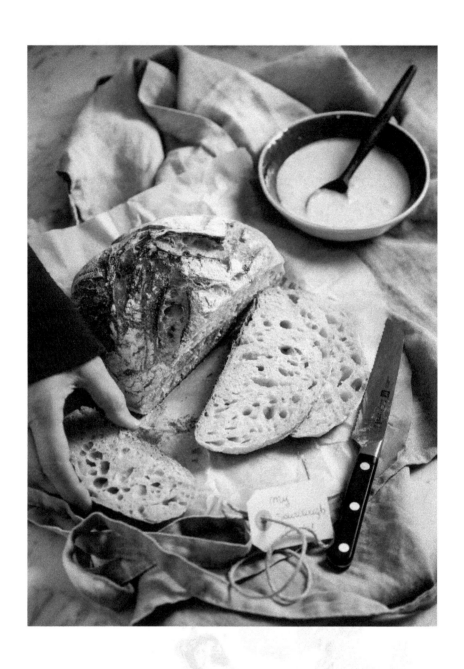

MEDITERRANEAN
APPETIZERS

Roasted Balsamic Beets

Total time: 1 hour 30 minutes

Prep time: 15 minutes

Cook time: 1 hour 15 minutes

Yields: 4 servings

Ingredients

- 3-4 medium beets
- 2 tbsp. extra virgin olive oil
- 1 tbsp. balsamic vinegar
- ½ tsp. sea salt

Directions

- Scrub the beets and wash well; cut into 6 wedges and place them in a baking dish.
- Drizzle the beets with extra virgin olive oil, vinegar, and salt and bake, covered, at 375°F for about 1 hour.
- Uncover and continue baking for 15 more minutes or until almost tender.

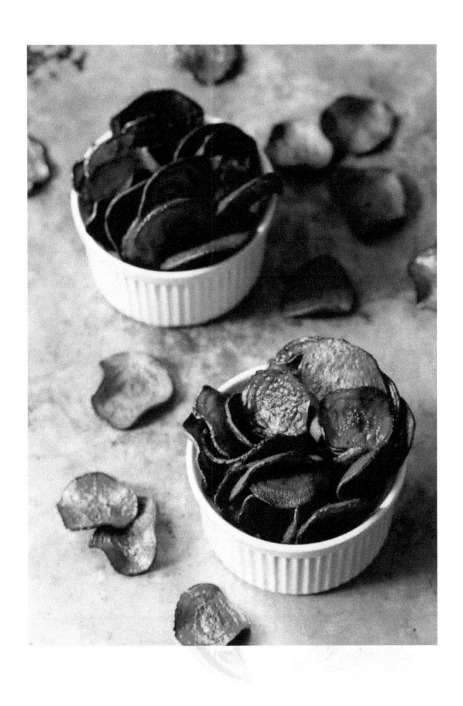

Fig Tapenade

Total time: 15 minutes

Prep time: 15 minutes

Cook time: 0 minutes

Yields: 16 servings

Ingredients

- 1 cup dried figs
- ½ cup water
- 1 cup Kalamata olives
- 1 tbsp. chopped fresh thyme
- ½ tsp. balsamic vinegar
- 1 tbsp. extra virgin olive oil

Directions

- Pulse the figs in a food processor until well chopped; add water and continue pulsing to form a paste. Add olives and pulse until well blended.
- Add thyme, vinegar, and extra virgin olive oil and pulse until very smooth.
- Serve with walnut crackers.